Essential Oils Vitality Guide

33 Advanced Aromatherapy Tips and Tricks for Weight Loss, Stress Relief And Anti-Aging

Introduction

I want to thank you and congratulate you for purchasing the book, *"Essential Oils Vitality Guide: 33 Advanced Aromatherapy Tips and Tricks for Weight Loss, Stress Relief and Anti-Aging"*.

This book contains proven steps and strategies on how to effectively address common daily concerns such as weight gain, stress, and aging using the wonders of essential oils.

If you are struggling with any of the issues above, I wrote this book to provide you with alternative techniques in the essential oil therapy realm that could have a huge impact on your well-being. They are not the end-all for self improvement, weight loss, or even anti-aging, but they can play a very vital role in getting you to where you want to go with any of those areas.

I truly hope the techniques and special essential oil blends listed in this book will help you revitalize your health as well as help you jump-start your day to feel renewed and refreshed.

Thanks again for purchasing this book, I hope you enjoy it!

Chapter 1 - Understanding Essential Oil Therapy

Over the years, people have had the common notion of "aromatherapy" as anything that smells good, like scented candles and perfumes. Aromatherapy, in fact, is defined as the therapeutic application of plant essential oils (usually diluted in some type of solution) by qualified individuals. There has been a bit of a misnomer because the word aromatherapy suggests that all essential oils smell nice. On the contrary, a number of essential oils do not have a satisfactory scent. Therefore, essential oil therapy, ideally is the more descriptive name for this topic.

Currently, there is a growing body of research focused on the remarkable healing properties of essential oils. The definition of the term essential oil is that it is a natural compound extracted from the stems, leaves, fruits, roots, and/or flowers of one particular plant species. These are referred to as oils mainly because they are composed of the oil-soluble chemicals in the plant (usually 100 to 200 chemicals per essential oil), not because they have an oily texture. The properties that make essential oils therapeutic are derived from its complex chemistry. Oils from the exact same plant but extracted using different methods will actually reveal varying results. There are multiple methods to extract an essential oil from one plant. The two common methods include steam distillation, and expression. Based on the plant's chemical make-up, one method may be more fitting for specific plants than others.

Steam distillation is the method by which the most pure essential oil extracts are derived from plants. Steam is made to pass through the newly harvested plant material, causing the lighter chemicals contained within it to vaporize. The steam is collected in a vessel, travels through a tubing, and finally condenses through a cooling process. The two products generated in this process are the oil-soluble essential oil, and the water-soluble hydrosol or hydrolat. Since it is impossible for water and oil to mix, the two would naturally divide, and the essential oil is collected.

Expression is the most direct method of extracting essential oils from the plant's flesh, skins and seeds. The method is used mostly with citrus fruits, especially lemon, lime, grapefruit, and orange,. The procedure involves grating or scraping the peel of a citrus fruit to express the oils. For instance, when zesting a lemon, one should take great care so as to capture the volatile oils that would be expressed during the process. Heat is not a requirement in this process. It is for this reason that the chemistry of citrus essential oils is not heat-altered and the smell remains very similar to the fruits from which they come.

Newer extraction methods are currently becoming more common. One of the most interesting processes, although quite costly, is the super-critical carbon dioxide (CO_2) extraction. In this technique, the solvent that would be utilized is carbon dioxide, which is included and then eliminated to produce a high-grade extract with an essential oil scent that is very close to the plant itself. Compared to distilled oils, CO_2 extracts contain a wider range of the chemical molecules found in the plant material because less heat is used and some different components are absorbed by CO_2 extraction.

Other older methods are worth mentioning. Enfleurage is quite an ancient method. With the exception of France, it is no longer commonly used today because of its long and complicated process that has become very expensive. Sheets of animal fat or vegetable fat absorb the oil from the blossoms. The old blossoms are replaced several times with fresh ones until the fat is infused with fragrance. This can take a lot of time, from days to weeks. The fat is then washed with solvents, separating just the essential oil.

Essential oils can also be extracted through chemical solvents. However, this technique is not commonly used by most aromatherapists nowadays because they worry that slight traces of the solvent may remain even though they are supposed to be completely removed. The process includes dissolving the plant in a solvent such as chlorure of benzene, methylene, or hexane. The solvent, having a low boiling point, is then evaporated off to pull it away from the essential oil. The product oils are referred to as the absolutes. When paraffin waxes are used as solvents, the remaining paraffins cause the final results to become solidified, and thus it is called "concrete. This method is expensive and reserved for costly oils that cannot be distilled, such as in the case of vanilla and jasmine. Essential oil from the rose is also extracted through this technique because it is slightly less expensive when obtained through this process rather than through distillation.

Depending on the way the essential oil is produced the quality and concentration can be highly affected. And because they are derived from nature, the specific species of plant, how it was grown, how the oils were extracted and stored, and the kind of soil conditions (cloud cover, the type of soil, and the temperature) all have effects on the quality of an essential oil. There are three major characteristics that influence the quality of an essential oil, and these are grade, purity, and integrity.

Grades

Different processing techniques can produce different essential oil grades. For instance, re-distillation of peppermint produces oil that is stronger than other substances, so the chewing gum and candy that it adds flavor to has a less strong and fresher taste and scent. Those with higher grades costs twice compared to the ones with the lesser grades. Higher grades generally are more intense and carry a richer bouquet of fragrance. The oils with lower quality are usually still pure essential oil, but the scent is less potent or even weak because of the lower range of the aromatic compounds.

At times, two bottles of the same kind of oil smell differently. This does not necessarily mean that one is better than the other. For instance, one geranium essential oil may carry a noticeably stronger hint of citrus while another smells more like rose. Most people will prefer using the rose because of its scent, but in truth there is not much of a difference.

Purity

Purity is an important concern to anyone purchasing essential oils because they can be contaminated or entirely replaced with a cheaper substitute or extended or diluted with vegetable oils, alcohol, or solvents. These substitutes and extenders lessen the potency of the oil. Alteration is not common in cheaper oils such as peppermint, orange, or cedar but more common with the pricier oils that are in great demand, such as melissa, jasmine, and rose. Even if a product is labeled as pure essential oil, it is not often the case. For instance, an oil that is labeled as vanilla or rose may have been produced in a company not from natural ingredients but actually from synthetic chemicals. However, these can still be labeled as essential oils.

Integrity

Integrity means that the oil is pure and natural and not whipped up in a laboratory or composed of cheaper essential oil substitutes. It should come from a single species of plant (and probably even from the same region and harvest). Inexpensive citronella or lemongrass essential oils are sometimes used to disguise as the very expensive melissa (lemon balm) oil. Rose essential oils are artificially made in the laboratory by using rose germanium then chemically altering it to mimic a rose scent. The problem here is that although the end product still contains only pure, natural essential oils, it never completely accurately copies the real thing.

Most essential oils are safe and free of adverse side effects when used properly. However, it is important to determine the quality of essential oils as there can be a big difference between what a professional aromatherapist would use and what is sold in the retail and health stores. On your own, you will not be able to spot them simply by looking. But in order to achieve maximum healing benefits from aromatherapy treatments, using a premium quality oil is of the essence.

Chapter 2 - Carrier Oils, Essential Oils and Blends

Carrier oils come from the kernels, seeds, and flesh of various plants. These oils serve as vessels that deliver the essential oil properties over the surface of the skin, which would then enable absorption. Along with the benefits of essential oils, you also absorb the vitamins and individual properties of the carrier oil. It is also known as base oil or vegetable oil. The following lists the best-known and most readily available carrier oils:

- Sweet Almond Oil (*Prunus dulcis*)
- Apricot Kernel Oil (*Prunus armeniaca*)
- Avocado Oil (*Persea americana*)
- Canola Oil (*Brassica napus L or Brassica campestris L or Brassica rapa var*):
- Cocoa Butter (*Theobroma cacao*)
- Coconut Oil Fractionated (*Cocos nucifera*)
- Grapeseed Oil (*Vitus vinifera*)
- Hazelnut Oil (*Vitus vinifera*)
- Jojoba (*Simmondsia chinensis*)
- Kukui Nut Oil (*Aleurites moluccans*)
- Olive Oil (*Olea europaea*)
- Shea Butter (*Butyrospermum parkii*)
- Sunflower Oil (*Helianthus annuus*)

Comprehensive List of Essential Oils:
Research on each oil from a reputable online source before use:
- Allspice (*Pimenta officinalis*)
- Amyris (*Amyris balsamifera*)
- Angelica root (*Angelica officinalis*)
- Anise (*Pimpinella anisum*)
- Basil (*Ocimum basilicum*)
- Bergamot (*Citrus bergamia*)
- Cajeput (*Melaleuca cajeputi*)
- Camphor, white (*Cinnamonum camphora*)

- Cardamom (*Elletaria cardamomum*)
- Carrot seed (*Daucus carota*)
- Chamomile, Roman (*Anthemis nobilis*)
- Chamomile, German (*Matricaria chamomilla*)
- Cinnamon leaf (*Cinnamomum zeylancium*)
- Clove bud (*Eugenia caryophyllata*)
- Citronella (*Cymbopogon nardus*)
- Clary sage (*Salvia sclarea*)
- Coriander (*Coriandrum sativum*)
- Cypress (*Cupressus sempervirens*)
- *Eucalyptus globulus*
- *Eucalyptus radiata*
- Fennel (*Foeniculum vulgare var. dulce*)
- Frankincense (*Boswellia frereana*)
- Galbanum (*Ferula galbaniflua*)
- Ginger (*Zingiber officinale*)
- Grapefruit (*Citrus paradisi*)
- Geranium (*Pelargonium graveolens*)
- Helichrysum (*Helichrysum italicum*)
- Juniper berry (*Juniperus communis*)
- Jasmine absolute (*Jasminum grandiflorum*)
- Lemon (*Citrus limonum*)
- Lemongrass (*Cymbopogon citratus*)
- Lavender (*Lavandula angustifolia*)
- Lime (*Citrus aurantifolia*)
- Litsea (*Litsea cubeba*)
- Marjoram (*Origanum marjorana*)
- Melissa (*Melissa officinalis*)
- Mandarin (*Citrus reticulata*)
- Myrrh (*Commiphora myrrha*)
- Neroli (*Citrus aurantium var. amara*)
- Nutmeg (*Myristica fragrans*)
- Orange, sweet (*Citrus sinensis*)
- Patchouli (*Pogostemon cablin*)
- Pepper, black (*Piper nigrum*)
- Petitgrain (*Citrus aurantium*)
- Peppermint (*Mentha piperita*)

- Pine (*Pinus sylvestris*)
- Palmarosa (*Cymbopogon martini*)
- Ravensara (*Ravensara aromatica*)
- Rosemary (*Rosmarinus officinalis*)
- Rose (*Rosa damascena*)
- Spearmint (*Mentha spicata*)
- Sandalwood (*Santalum album*)
- Vetiver (*Vetiveria zizanioides*)
- Tea tree (*Melaleuca alternifolia*)
- Ylang ylang (*Cananga odorata*)

Creating Essential Oil Blends

In creating your perfect blend of essential oils it is imperative to note three aspects. First of all, you need to know exactly what you want to accomplish. Secondly, you must be knowledgeable about every essential oil and how they are used. Then, you should only choose 100 percent (pure) essential oils.

The "aesthetic essential oil blend" focuses on beauty and fragrance. It has very little to do with the therapeutic properties of the essential oil. These blends are created for perfumes or to mist the room.

On a different note, the "therapeutic aromatherapy blend" is all about application of the healing properties of the essential oils whether in acute or in chronic concerns. Research needs to be conducted for you to be knowledgeable about the benefits of the essential oils and your health and lifestyle conditions (sleep pattern, eating habits, medical issues, and so on). Concocting a blend requires careful consideration of all the possible essential oils that would suit specific health conditions before you can come up with your combination that is just right for you.

Bath Oil Recipe

A few drops of skin-safe essential oils can be added directly to bathwater, but it is better to add a carrier oil such as what is suggested in this recipe for it to minimize skin sensitivity and help to moisturize and nourish your skin.

Ingredients:
- 2 fl ounces carrier oil of your choice
- 20 drops of your preferred essential oil blend (such as Lavender)

Directions: combine the oils and transfer into a glass or plastic container, seal tightly, and place in your refrigerator.

To Use: Do not use all 2 fl ounces of bath oil for each bath. Do not use more than ¼ fl ounce of the bath oil blend to the bathwater just before getting into the water. Combine thoroughly by mixing the blend into the bath water with your hand to ensure that the oil is thoroughly combined.

Bath Salt Recipe

Ingredients:
- 3 cups salt. Recommended salt types: Sea Salt, Himalayan Pink Salt, Epsom salt, Dead Sea Salt
- 17 to 24 drops of your preferred essential oil or essential oil blend

Optional: 1 tablespoon carrier oil, such as Jojoba

Directions: Place the salts into a bowl. Use a spoon or fork to combine. Mix in the measured amount of the essential oils and combine. Spoon the blend into an airtight container to make sure that the scent does not evaporate. Disturb the contents in the container everyday to ensure that the oils are well combined.

To Use: Add less than 1 cup of the bath salts just before you place yourself inside the tub. Combine thoroughly to ensure that the bath salt has dissolved and melted into the bathwater before use. Otherwise, you would end up sitting uncomfortably on bits of chunky salts.

Massage Oil Recipe

Ingredients:
- 1 fl ounce carrier oil, such as Sweet Almond Oil
- 10 to 12 drops of your desired essential oils

Directions: Combine the oils well and transfer to a tightly sealed dark glass container.

To Use: Place only a tiny amount on the skin and massage.

Room Mist Air Freshener Recipe

Ingredients:
- 4 oz. clean spray bottle
- 30 drops of your prefered essential oil or essential oil blend
- 1.5 fl ounces of distilled water or hydrosol

1.5 fl ounces of high-proof alcohol (do not use isopropyl or rubbing alcohol).

Recommended Essential Oils:
- 4 drops Ylang Ylang
- 20 drops Lime
- 14 drops Bergamot
- 2 drops Rose
- 4 drops Peppermint
- 9 drops Lemon
- 6 drops Lavender
- 20 drops Rosemary
- 15 drops Clary Sage
- 8 drops Grapefruit
- 2 drops Spearmint (optional)

Directions: Fill the 4 oz. spray bottle with pure distilled water or with alcohol and distilled water. Mix in the desired essential oil or blend. Seal, shake and start spraying. After 24 hours, you can check the room to see if the potency of the scent is strong enough, otherwise adjust contents based on the results.

To Use: Shake the contents of the bottle very well before using each time.

Chapter 3 - Aromatherapy for Weight Loss

The use of essential oils alone will certainly be enough to help you with weight loss. However, if you are already following an effective weight loss plan, the use of essential oils will further boost your chances of achieving your desired weight loss results. Make sure to talk to a medical professional, including a nutritionist, before engaging in an form of weight loss program so that you can tailor-fit it to your personal medical concerns. There are multiple causes for one to gain weight, including medical and physical concerns, a sedentary lifestyle, not being knowledgeable about the importance of nutrition, emotional eating, not being conscious of when, where, and what you eat, and a host of other factors such as grief and depression.

Such factors can be addressed with the help of aromatherapy, especially if you choose specific essential oils that can help strengthen your concentration, improve your willpower, and boost your energy. These will help you remain disciplined and determined to follow your weight loss program. Also, the use of essential oils can help you avoid food cravings, boost your metabolism, improve your digestive system functions, regulate your blood sugar levels, and boost your mood. Therefore, aromatherapy is part of a holistic approach towards weight loss once it is combined with a healthy diet, regular workout routines, and other healthy habits.

Grapefruit Blend for Weight Loss

Drink: Add 1 to 2 drops of grapefruit essential oil (food grade) to one glass of water. Drink it first thing when you wake up in the morning.

Massage Oil: Add a few drops of grapefruit essential oil to olive oil. Then, massage on to the area for 30 minutes where fat accumulates.

Lemon Blend for Weight Loss

Inhalation: Add a few drops of lemon essential oil to a cotton ball. Slowly breathe in the essence before a meal to help reduce your appetite.

Drink: Add 1 to 2 drops of lemon essential oil (food grade) to one glass of water. Drink it first thing in the morning to help your body startup digestion and detoxification.

Massage Oil: Add a few drops of lemon essential oil to your favorite carrier oil. Then massage the area where fat or cellulite accumulates to detoxify fat cells.

Peppermint Blend for Weight Loss

Inhalation: Add a few drops of peppermint essential oil to a cotton ball. Slowly breathe in the essence before a meal to help reduce your appetite.

Drink: Add 1 to 2 drops of peppermint essential oil (food grade) to one glass of water. Drink before a meal to reduce appetite and avoid overeating.

Bath Oil: Add 5 to 10 drops of peppermint essential oil to your morning bath to energize your body and reduce food cravings.

Cinnamon Blend for Weight Loss

Drink: Add 1 to 2 drops of cinnamon essential oil (food grade) to a cup of warm water with a little honey. Drink it before each meal to reduce your appetite or prior to bedtime to avoid midnight cravings.

Inhalation: Put a few droplets of cinnamon essential oil to a cotton ball. Slowly breathe in the essence before a meal.

Bergamot Blend for Weight Loss

Inhalation: Add a few drops of bergamot essential oil on a cloth. Slowly breathe in the essence boost your mood and give you an overall relaxing effect. Do this when you find yourself looking for comfort food.

Feet or Neck Rub: Dilute a few drops of bergamot essential oil in olive or coconut oil. Lightly rub on the feet and neck to wind down.

Bath Oil: Dilute a few drops of bergamot essential oil in olive or coconut oil. Mix in a couple of drops to your bath to help you through the day in controlling your food cravings when stressed or emotional.

Goodbye Cellulite Bath Blend

Ingredients:

- 5 drops Lemon
- 5 drops Grapefruit
- 5 drops Sandalwood
- 5 drops Ginger
- 5 drops Orange
- 1 cup Raw Apple Cider Vinegar

Directions: Add 5 drops of each essential oil to 1 cup raw apple cider vinegar. Mix the blend into the warm water for your bath just before getting in the tub. Mix well by splashing it around your hand through the bathwater. Soak yourself for at about half an hour.

Weight Loss in a Capsule

Ingredients:

- 2 drops Peppermint
- 2 drops Grapefruit
- 2 drops Lemon
- 12 drops Coconut oil (liquefied)

Directions: Combine 2 drops of each essential oil in a dark colored bottle. Mix in the measured drops of coconut oil. Transfer the blend into a capsule. You can choose to double the recipe to if you want to prepare multiple capsules. Store the capsules in a cool place. Take one capsule per day.

Chapter 4 - Aromatherapy for Stress Relief

Essential oils have the capacity to directly access the brain's limbic system, the part of the brain linked to memory and emotions. They may be used to create a positive emotional state, create an environment of relaxation at the end of a long day, help soothe grief or worries, and a lot more.

Rest and Relaxation Aromatherapy

Your work and demands of daily life can bring about chronic stress, resulting in health issues such as poor digestion, insomnia, increase in weight, nausea, etc. Your busy schedule makes it difficult for you to find time to relax, however, try our pure, relaxing blend and you will find yourself pampered to the soul.

Ingredients:

- 1 fl ounce Sweet Almond Oil
- 7 drops Roman Chamomile
- 5 drops Lavender

Directions:

Massage Oil: Mix the oils very well place in an air-tight, clean, dark glass container. Massage it gently into your feet or let someone give you a foot massage for a more delightful experience. Roman Chamomile has a strong soothing properties effect, so make sure you have no plans of driving after.

Diffuser Blend: Adjust the blend to a ratio of 2 drops Roman Chamomile to 1 drop Lavender. Then, add to your diffuser.

Aromatherapy for Energy and Alertness

A busy-bee? Try these blends to help you get through you daily hectic schedule.

Option 1   2 drops Grapefruit, 1 drop Cypress, 2 drops Basil

Option 2   2 drops Ginger, 3 drops Grapefruit

Option 3   2 drops Rosemary, 3 drops Bergamot

Option 4   2 drops Peppermint, 2 drops Lemon, 1 drop Frankincense

Directions:

Diffuser Blend: The blend may be quadrupled to obtain a total of twenty drops of your blend of choice. Transfer the oils to a tightly sealed, deep colored glass container and combine thoroughly by rolling it between your palms. Then, mix in the correct number of drops of your created blend to your diffuser as provided in the user instructions.

Bath Oil: Triple the blend and continue by following the instructions provided in Bath Oil Recipe.

Bath Salts: Quadruple the blend and continue by following the instructions provided in Bath Salts Recipes.

Massage Oil: Double the amount used and simply follow the same instructions in the Massage Oil Recipes.

Air Freshener: Multiply your blend by six. Then, proceed to the Room Mist Air Freshener Recipe and follow the same steps.

Aromatherapy for a Restful Sleep

Having difficulty in achieving a tranquil and restful night of rest? Aromatherapy may not be the only cure for symptoms of insomnia, but this blend may be able to help ease your mind and body, and could even enable you to fall asleep more quickly. The next day, you would even experience feeling bright eyed and bushy tailed.

Ingredients:

- 3 drops Lavender
- 1 drop Chamomile
- 1 drop Clary Sage

Directions: First, take off the casing of your pillow. Add the suggested number of drops onto a cotton ball. Then use the cotton ball to apply the mixture onto the surface of the pillow. Set aside for several minutes before you slip the pillow back into the pillowcase. Do not attempt to add the essential oils directly on your pillowcase as this might cause eye and skin irritation while you sleep due to your direct contact with the oils. If you do not want to add the oils to your pillow, an alternative would be to inhale the blend of oils from the cotton ball before you go to sleep.

Aromatherapy for Anger

Do you always find it difficult to manage your anger? These essential oils can help bring calm during intense times.

Option 1   1 drop Vetiver, 1 drop Rose, 3 drops Orange

Option 2   3 drops Bergamot, 1 drop Jasmine, 1 drop Ylang Ylang

Option 3   2 drops Bergamot, 1 drop Roman Chamomile, 2 drops Orange

Option 4   2 drops Patchouli, 3 drops Orange

Directions: May be experienced as a bath oil, diffused blend, massage oil, air freshener or bath salt by using the same steps as seen in the "Aromatherapy for Energy and Alertness" blend directions.

Aromatherapy for Anxiety

Option 1   1 drop Frankincense, 2 drops Bergamot, 2 drops Clary Sage
Option 2   2 drops Bergamot, 3 drops Sandalwood
Option 3   2 drops Clary Sage, 3 drops Lavender
Option 4   1 drop Rose, 1 drop Lavender, 1 drop Vetiver, 2 drops Mandarin

Directions: May be experienced as a bath oil, diffused blend, massage oil, air freshener or bath salt by using the same steps as seen in the "Aromatherapy for Energy and Alertness" blend directions.

Aromatherapy to Enhance Happiness

These blends can help you feel joyful and relaxed. Citrus oils are a great way for when you are seeking a pleasant and happy environment.

Option 1   1 drop Grapefruit, 1 drop Ylang Ylang, 3 drops Bergamot
Option 2   2 drops Frankincense, 1 drop Geranium, 2 drops Orange
Option 3   1 drop Rose, 2 drops Sandalwood, 2 drops Bergamot
Option 4   1 drop Rose or Neroli, Ylang Ylang, Orange or Bergamot, 2 drops Lemon, 2 drops Grapefruit

Directions: May be experienced as a bath oil, diffused blend, massage oil, air freshener or bath salt by using the same steps as seen in the "Aromatherapy for Energy and Alertness" blend directions.

Aromatherapy to Help Boost Confidence

These essential oil blends has the power to influence your mental state. They are made to enable you to unleash your strengths and support your mental energy.

Option 1   2 drops Bay Laurel, 3 drops Bergamot
Option 2   2 drops Rosemary, 3 drops Orange
Option 3   1 drop Jasmine, 4 drops Bergamot
Option 4   2 drops Cypress, 3 drops Grapefruit

Directions: May be experienced as a bath oil, diffused blend, massage oil, air freshener or bath salt by using the same steps as seen in the "Aromatherapy for Energy and Alertness" blend directions.

Aromatherapy to Ease Feelings of Panic Attacks

Option 1   3 drops Frankincense, 2 drops Helichrysum

Option 2   4 drops Lavender, 1 drop Rose

Option 3   4 drops Lavender, 1 drop Neroli

Option 4   1 drop Rose, 4 drops Frankincense

Directions: May be experienced as a bath oil, diffused blend, massage oil, air freshener or bath salt by using the same steps as seen in the "Aromatherapy for Energy and Alertness" blend directions.

Aromatherapy to Minimize Irritability

Option 1   2 drops Lavender, 3 drops Mandarin

Option 2   1 drop Neroli, 2 drops Lavender, 2 drops Roman Chamomile

Option 3   1 drop Neroli, 4 drops Sandalwood

Option 4   3 drops Sandalwood, 2 drops Mandarin

Option 5   2 drops Mandarin, 3 drops Roman Chamomile

Directions: May be experienced as a bath oil, diffused blend, massage oil, air freshener or bath salt by using the same steps as seen in the "Aromatherapy for Energy and Alertness" blend directions.

Aromatherapy for Depression

Option 1   1 drop Orange, 1 drop Rose, 3 drops Sandalwood

Option 2   2 drops Clary Sage, 3 drops Bergamot

Option 3   3 drops Grapefruit, 1 drop Ylang Ylang, 1 drop Lavender

Option 4   1 drop Lemon, 2 drops Frankincense, 2 drops Jasmine
or Neroli

Directions: May be experienced as a bath oil, diffused blend, massage oil, air freshener or bath salt by using the same steps as seen in the "Aromatherapy for Energy and Alertness" blend directions.

Aromatherapy to Ease Loneliness

Option 1   1 drop Rose, 2 drops Frankincense, 2 drops Bergamot

Option 2   3 drops Clary Sage, 2 drops Bergamot

Option 3   3 drops Bergamot, 2 drops Roman Chamomile

Option 4   3 drops Clary Sage, 2 drops Frankincense

Directions: May be experienced as a bath oil, diffused blend, massage oil, air freshener or bath salt by using the same steps as seen in the "Aromatherapy for Energy and Alertness" blend directions.

Aromatherapy to Ease Insecurity

Option 1   1 drop Vetiver, 1 drop Jasmine, 3 drops Bergamot,

Option 2   2 drops Cedarwood, 2 drops Bergamot, 1 drop Frankincense

Option 3   4 drops Sandalwood, 1 drop Jasmine

Option 4   3 drops Sandalwood, 2 drops Frankincense

Directions: May be experienced as a bath oil, diffused blend, massage oil, air freshener or bath salt by using the same steps as seen in the "Aromatherapy for Energy and Alertness" blend directions.

Chapter 5 - Aromatherapy for Anti-Aging

For thousands of years, use of essential oils has been an important element in women's daily beauty regimen. They are essential in soothing away the appearance of fine lines and wrinkles, visible signs of aging, and restoring a radiant-looking complexion. Rediscover your natural beauty with these blends:

Exfoliating Sugar Scrub 1
Ingredients:
- 11 net wt. oz. Melt & Pour Soap Base
- 2 cups White Sugar
- 4 fl ounce cold pressed Vegetable Oil such as Watermelon Seed Oil, Jojoba or Fractionated Coconut Oil
- 1/4 tsp Vitamin E Oil (1400 IU is Ideal)
- 1/4 fl ounce (1.5 tsp.) Essential Oil

Directions: Gently melt (without overheating) the Melt & Pour Soap Base until it is completely melted using the double-boiler. Then immediately pour it into a mixing bowl. Add the vegetable oils and Vitamin E Oil and quickly stir to combine. Add sugar while continuously stirring. Add the essential oil and mix well. Add more sugar if your mixture is too thin. Pack the mixture into your soap mold and press firmly to prevent air pockets. Allow to set for an hour. Unmold the scrubs before the mixture is completely set to make it easier to cut the cubes. Cut into approximately 1-inch cubes. Allow to firm up at room temperature for several hours.

To Use: The scrub cubes can be used on the body and feet, but avoid using it on the face. Use one cube each time you need to exfoliate. Simply take one with you each time you enter the shower. Allow it to get wet, and massage the cube into a soft workable, exfoliating paste in the palm of your hand. Scrub gently in a slow, circular motion. Do not rub the scrub deeply onto your skin. Rinse off. Moisturize the skin with a natural moisturizer after exfoliating.

Exfoliating Sugar Scrub 2
Ingredients:
- 8 net wt. ounces Turbinado Sugar or Demerara Sugar
- 1 fl ounce cold pressed Vegetable Oil such as Fractionated Coconut Oil, Jojoba or Watermelon Seed Oil

or
- 1 fl oz Vegetable Glycerin
- 1 fl oz Liquid Castille Soap
- 1/2 tsp Vitamin E Oil (1400 IU is Ideal)
- 1/4 tsp Essential Oil

Directions: Using a small- to medium-sized mixing bowl, put the sugar into it. Then, add the oils, glycerin and castille soap to the bowl and mix well with a fork. Lastly, add the essential oil and mix thoroughly.

To Use: This scrub can be used on the face or body. Scoop a small amount of the scrub onto your fingers and transfer it onto wet skin. Lightly rub in gentle, circular movements without grinding onto your skin. Rinse off. If desired, follow with gentle cleansing and moisturize after exfoliating.

Aromatherapy for Arthritis

Stay young and active! Support your bones and joints with these blends to help you maintain movement and vitality.

Option 1: 2 fl ounces Carrier Oil such as Jojoba, 20 drops Roman Chamomile, 4 drops Black Pepper

Option 2: 2 fl ounces Carrier Oil such as Jojoba, 10 drops Roman Chamomile, 10 drops Helichrysum

Directions: Select your blend and mix all oils together. Store in an airtight, dark-colored glass jar. Lightly rub onto arthritic joints but only use a small amount of the blend.

Mega Anti-Aging Serum

Ingredients:
- 1/2 cup Apricot Kernel Oil
- 10 drops Carrot Seed Oil
- 10 drops Rose Hip Seed
- 5 drops Geranium
- 5 drops Lemon
- 10 drops Sandalwood
- 5 drops Frankincense
- 5 drops Myrrh
- 5 drops Rosemary

Directions: Add ½ cup Apricot Kernel Oil in a 4 oz amber jar. Then add drops of essential oils. With a dropper, apply an amount that is approximately one teaspoon on your hand and rub into your face and neck. Do this after you have cleansed your face at night.

Natural Anti-Oxidant Serum

As we age, our bodies take on more insults from cell-damaging free radicals. Working out and eating the right types of food, while essential to good health, might not be enough to make you look and feel younger. Get help by using this blend.

Ingredients:
- 1/2 cup Apricot Kernel Oil
- 10 drops Carrot Seed
- 10 drops Rosehip Seed

Directions: Combine all oils in an amber bottle. Then, rub a small amount into face and neck after cleansing.

Skin Firming and Age Reversal Skin Serum

Ingredients:
- 2 tbsp Rosehip Seed Oil
- 2 tbsp Sweet Almond Oil
- 10 drops Cypress
- 10 drops Geranium
- 7 drops Frankincense

Directions: Combine all oils in an amber bottle. Then, rub a small amount into face and neck after cleansing.

No More Scars Blend

Use apricot kernel and rosehip as carrier oils (or some other combination) and as many of the following essential oils as you desire.

Ingredients:
- 1 fl ounce Rosehip Seed Oil
- 1 fl ounce Apricot Kernel Oil
- 5 drops Helichrysum
- 5 drops Carrot Seed
- 5 drops Frankincense
- 5 drops Calendula
- 5 drops Rosemary
- 10 Drops Lavender

Directions: Combine all the oils and apply directly to scar twice daily.

Shea Butter Sunblock

Ingredients:
- 1/2 cup Shea Butter
- 1/3 cup Coconut Oil (melted)
- 15 drops Carrot Seed
- 10 drops Myrrh
- 2 tbsp zinc oxide (optional)

Directions: Whip shea butter in a bowl until creamy. Slowly add the melted coconut oil while whipping. Add essential oils until fluffy. Do not inhale when adding zinc oxide.

Note:

SPF: 40+ (with zinc oxide)

SPF: 20-30 (without zinc oxide)

Sunscreen Oil

Ingredients:
- 1/2 cup Fractionated Coconut Oil
- 10 drops Myrrh (add up to 40 drops for higher SPF)
- 5 drops Carrot Seed

Directions: Combine all the oils and store in an amber-colored jar. Apply over exposed areas of the skin. Reapply as needed.

Aloe Vera Sunblock

Ingredients:
- 1 cup Aloe Vera Juice
- ¼ cup Avocado Oil
- 15 drops Carrot Seed
- 10 drops Myrrh

Directions: Add all the oils in a sprayer bottle. Shake well before every use.

Anti-Aging Facial Toner

Ingredients:
- 1 fl ounce High Proof Vodka
- 2.5 fl ounce Witch Hazel Hydrosol
- 8 drops Grapefruit
- 4 drops Tea Tree
- 4 drops Cypress

Directions: Add all ingredients in a 4 oz. bottle and shake to mix well. The 0.5 oz. unfilled space in the bottle allows room for reshaking the toner before each use to disperse the essential oils. Apply to your face using a cotton ball.

Detox Face Mask Recipe

Ingredients:
- 1 tbsp Bentonite Clay
- 1 tsp Activated Charcoal
- 2 tbsp Raw Honey
- 2 tbsp Aloe Vera Gel
- 3 tbsp Grapeseed
- 5-6 drops Essential Oil of choice

Directions: Combine all ingredients in a non-metal container and stir with a wooden or plastic spoon. Massage onto face and neck. Leave it on for 15 to 20 minutes and then rinse with warm water.

Acne Spot Treatment

Ingredients:
- 1 fl ounce Jojoba or Fractionated Coconut Oil
- 6 drops Lavender

- 5 drops Tea Tree
- 1 drop Geranium

Directions: Pour the selected carrier oil into a very clean amber-colored bottle. Add the essential oils and tightly close the bottle. Roll the bottle between your palms for a minute or two to properly mix the oils. Apply a small amount to the face, neck or back after cleansing. Use once daily as needed. Gently roll the bottle before each use.

Bees Wax Sunblock

Ingredients:
- ¼ cup Avocado Oil
- ¼ cup Coconut Oil
- ¼ cup Beeswax
- ¼ cup Shea Butter
- 10 drops Myrrh
- 15 drops Carrot Seed
- 2 tbsp Zinc oxide (optional or you can add more myrrh up to 40 drops)

Directions: Using a double broiler, add the avocado oil, coconut oil and beeswax. Stir on low heat until. When the oils have melted, remove from heat to add shea butter and the essential oils. Stir until shea butter is melted. Then, add zinc oxide if you choose to until there are no clumps. Transfer to a storage container, and use as your regular sunscreen.

Chapter 6 - How to Handle Essential Oils Safely

Keep all essential oils out of reach of children and pets. Many essential oils such as citrus oils can smell like they are "yummy" and safe to drink. If a child appears to have drunk several spoonfuls of an essential oil, rush to the nearest emergency center in your area or bring the child to the nearest health care center. Keep the bottle for identification and let the child drink whole or 2% milk. Do not try to induce vomiting.

It is not recommended to use photosensitizing essential oils before going under the sun or into a sun tanning booth. This can cause burning, redness, inflammation, and possibly several other forms of irritation when exposed to strong UVA rays. You should steer clear of the sun and refrain from using the sun tanning booth for at least twenty-four hours after treatment if photosensitizing essential oils were applied to the skin. Keep in mind that citrus oils are generally considered to be phototoxic.

Avoid the use of essential oils that you are not familiar with. Make sure to read up as much as you can about particular oils prior to using them. Not all essential oils are suitable for use in aromatherapy. Some are simply too toxic to use, including rue, pennyroyal, camphor (brown or yellow), horseradish, onion, wintergreen, bitter almond, mugwort, sassafras, calamus, mustard, buchu, savory, southerwood, tansy, wormseed, thuja, wormwood.

The rule of thumb is to never use undiluted essential oils on the skin. Essential oils can be mixed in with lotions, creams, shampoo, bath oil, bath salts, pure alcohol (to make perfume), body scrubs, and even room and body sprays. The only oils that can be used even if they are undiluted are lavender and tea tree, but with caution, as severe sensitivity could still occur in some individuals.

Perform a skin patch test on a small area of the skin if you suspect you may be sensitive to specific essential oils or if you have known allergies or sensitivities. If you notice any redness, burning or irritation, discontinue using the oil immediately and wash the area thoroughly with plain soap and water. If an essential oil triggers skin irritation, apply just a little bit of vegetable oil or cream to the affected area and discontinue use of the product.

Know the safety data on each essential oil and place into context of use and knowledge. Contraindications are meant to warn you of the side-effects of essential oils and are there to let you know which oils to avoid when you have asthma, low blood sugar, epilepsy, diabetes, hypertension, or with other health conditions.

Use caution with essential oils if you are pregnant or trying to get pregnant. Oils to stay away from during this time include peppermint, marjoram, bitter almond, hyssop, clove bud, juniper berry, thyme, sweet fennel, rosemary, clary sage, myrrh, rose, wintergreen, sage, basil.

Less is more. When using essential oils, use the smallest amount recommended that will get the job done. Don't use more because essential oils are very concentrated.

Keep essential oils away from the eyes. If essential oil droplets accidentally get into the eye (or eyes) a cotton cloth or similar should be saturated with fatty oils such as olive and sesame oils, and use it to clean off the essential oil on the closed lid. You should also immediately flush the eyes with cool water.

Essential oils contain substances that could catch fire easily and must be kept away from contact with flames, such as fire, candles, cigarettes, matches, and gas cookers. Some other precautionary measures that you should take are to make sure your room has good ventilation and not to internally use essential oils unless you have the proper training on the safety issues involved.

Conclusion

Thank you again for purchasing this book!

I hope this book was able to help you to become more knowledgeable on the properties and benefits of essential oils and how you can use them in your daily beauty regimen, weight loss program, and for other health concerns. Remember that essential oil therapy is not a panacea to more pressing medical concerns. It is still advisable to visit your physician.

The next step is to apply these tips and tricks onto your daily schedule and see the changes over time! Share your experience with friends and enjoy!

Finally, if you enjoyed this book, then I'd like to ask you for a favor, would you be kind enough to leave a review for this book on Amazon? It'd be greatly appreciated!

Thank you and good luck!

Keep reading for a free preview of my next book:

"Leptin Diet Cookbook: The Belly Fat Burnin' Recipe Book for Losing Weight FAST with the Leptin Diet"!

Chapter 1: Leptin Diet And Weight Loss

These days, the mere mention of a new diet often draws suspicious and questioning looks from most people. Unsurprisingly, of course, as there has been many a scam diet that's cropped up in the past years. Numerous weight loss pills and drinks have been marketed to be totally effective only to turn out bogus or even dangerous to one's health. So what makes the Leptin Diet different? Well, to begin with, it isn't one of those unorthodox fad diets or a supplement that you take before every meal. To put it simply, it is a smarter and healthier way of looking at the food you consume- it isn't about how much you eat, it's all about *when* you are eating it.

Time isn't usually a factor when it comes to most diets. After all, who pays attention to the hour that they eat? For most folks, losing weight means eating much less than what they normally do. While this method works, there are also certain risks involved often seen in cases wherein a person begins to overdo the diet. Some refrain from even touching food at all. But what if there is a way to lose weight without having to go through the trouble of counting calories? Instead, you only need to be more mindful of what and when you consume. By having more awareness when it comes to these things, you can gain more control over your body as well as your overall weight loss.

Now, let's talk a bit more about the science of this particular diet. There is a little known 16-Da adipokine molecule called Leptin and by understanding it better, you increase your chances of losing weight faster but in a healthier way. After all, it is one of the major hormones that is responsible for managing the overall balance of our body.

So how exactly does it help with weight loss?

- Controls excessive fat storage. Our body stores fat for many different reasons and in most cases, it does this as a precaution- just in case you end up going for days without food. See, if you go on a starvation diet, this sets off a trigger in your body wherein instead of burning any fat you consume for energy, it begins storing it for future use. Leptin can help you control what is stored into fat and what is used for energy. You can make sure that your body uses more of the fat for fuel so that you don't end up with any excesses in the areas you don't want them in.

- Suppresses food cravings. Considered by many dieters as the foremost challenge when it comes to losing weight, cravings can certainly be hard to overcome. This is especially if you're just starting out with the process and have been used to indulging yourself whenever the craving appears. Did you know that there are cases wherein people have reportedly experienced extreme mood swings while dieting simply because they've been craving certain food but can't have it? You wouldn't want to reach that point so let Leptin make things easier for you. The hormone itself is capable of suppressing any cravings; acting as a mediator when it comes to long-term energy regulation thus lowering your desire for food. After all, we only begin to crave these things whenever the body feels like its low on fuel. So by properly regulating the energy flow, we can go on for longer without feeling the need to stuff ourselves full.

To check out the rest of this book, head over to the nearest PC and visit the following link: http://www.books4everyone.com/leptin